Yoga for Older People

Improve flexibility and Balance for Seniors

Dr. Monica Haman

Copyright © by Dr. Monica Haman 2023. All rights reserved.

Before this document is duplicated or reproduced in any manner, the publisher's consent must be gained. Therefore, the contents within can neither be stored electronically, transferred, nor kept in a database. Neither in part nor full can the document be copied, scanned, faxed, or retained without approval from the publisher or creator.

Table of Contents

INTRODUCTION

CHAPTER ONE
Overview of Chair Yoga
Benefits of Chair Yoga for Older People

CHAPTER TWO
Getting Started
Safety Considerations
Equipment Needed
Setting Up Your Space

CHAPTER THREE
Breathing Techniques for Chair Yoga
Diaphragmatic Breathing
Ujjayi Breathing
Nadi Shodhana Breathing

CHAPTER FOUR
Basic Chair Yoga Poses
A. Seated Cat-Cow
B. Seated Downward Facing Dog
C. Seated Mountain Pose

D. Seated Forward Bend
E. Seated Twist
F. Seated Chair Pose
G. Seated Easy Pose
H. Seated Cobra Pose
I. Seated Eagle Pose
J. Seated Half Moon Pose
L. Seated Half Lord of the Fishes Pose
M. Seated Head-to-Knee Pose
N. Seated Wheel Pose
O. Seated Hand-to-Big-Toe Pose
P. Seated Sun Salutation

CHAPTER FIVE
Intermediate Chair Yoga Poses
A. Seated Warrior Pose
B. Seated Triangle Pose
C. Seated Half Lotus
D. Seated Chair Balance
E. Seated Camel Pose
F. Seated Crescent Pose
G. Seated Side Angle Pose
H. Seated Chair Bow Pose
I. Seated Chair Pigeon Pose

CHAPTER SIX
Advanced Chair Yoga Poses
A. Seated Tree Pose
B. Seated Warrior II
C. Seated Half Lord of the Fishes
D. Seated Head-to-Knee Pose
E. Seated Eagle Pose
F. Seated Half Handstand
G. Seated Crow Pose
H. Seated Wheel Pose
I. Seated Headstand
J. Seated Lotus Pose

CHAPTER SEVEN
Chair Yoga Sequences
A. Morning Sequence
B. Afternoon Sequence
C. Evening Sequence

CHAPTER EIGHT
Special Considerations
A. Modifying Poses for Limited Mobility
B. Adapting Poses for Specific Conditions
C. Incorporating Props

CHAPTER NINE
A. Summary of Benefits
B. Encouragement to Continue Practicing
C. The Importance of Making Health a Priority
D. Additional Sources of Information
E. The Final Thoughts

INTRODUCTION

As we age, our bodies change and things that were once easy, like moving and exercising, can become more challenging. It is a natural part of the passage of time, but that doesn't mean that our physical and mental well-being should be neglected. On the contrary, it is more important than ever to take an active interest in our health and well-being as we grow older.

It is natural for seniors to feel uncertain about how to maintain their physical and mental health in a way that is safe and effective. But, it is commendable that you, dear reader, have taken an interest in your well-being despite the passage of time.

This is where "Chair Yoga for Older People: Improve Flexibility and Balance for Seniors" by the experienced Dr. Haman comes in. This book is specifically designed to address the unique needs of older adults and to help them improve their flexibility, balance, and overall health. Whether you are a senior who is new to yoga or an experienced practitioner looking for modifications to suit your changing body, this book has everything you need to get started.

The book offers a wide range of chair yoga exercises that are suitable for seniors of all abilities. From basic stretches and poses to more advanced sequences, this book has something for everyone. The exercises have been specifically designed to be gentle and safe, but still challenging enough to bring about positive changes in the body. The book also includes modifications and variations to suit different levels of mobility, so you can be sure that your well-being always comes first.

But this book is not just about the physical benefits of yoga. The practice of yoga can also bring about improvements in mental health, including reducing stress and anxiety.

The book includes breathing techniques, relaxation exercises and even a sequence to do throughout the day so that the benefits of yoga can be enjoyed at any time. The practice of yoga is known to help reduce stress, anxiety, and depression, which are common issues among older adults. The techniques and practices in this book will not only help improve your physical health, but also your mental and emotional well-being, making it a holistic approach to maintaining a healthy lifestyle.

Also, the book also addresses common concerns that seniors may have when it comes to exercise, such as

balance issues, joint pain, and limited mobility. It includes modifications and variations that cater to these concerns, making it accessible and safe for seniors of all abilities to practice.

Exercise should be something that is enjoyable and that is why this book offers an incredibly wide variety to choose from. The book is designed to be easy to follow, with clear instructions to guide you through each exercise. So whether you have a few minutes to spare in the morning or a few hours in the evening, you will find something in this book that is perfect for you.

Overall, "Chair Yoga for Older People: Improve Flexibility and Balance for Seniors" is a comprehensive guide that is tailored to the unique needs of older adults. It is an invaluable resource for anyone looking to improve their physical and mental well-being through the practice of yoga. The book is not just about maintaining a healthy body, but also about maintaining a healthy mind and spirit, and it's an excellent way to stay active and engaged in life as you age.

CHAPTER ONE

Overview of Chair Yoga

The form of yoga known as "Chair Yoga" is performed either while the practitioner is sitting in a chair or with the assistance of a chair for support. This practice is especially helpful for elderly persons, who may have restricted mobility or difficulties with regular yoga positions.

However, this does not exclude them from benefiting from it. Chair yoga provides the same advantages as conventional yoga, such as enhanced flexibility, balance, and general well-being, but it does so while using the support and stability that a chair affords the practitioner.

The ancient Indian discipline of yoga is the origin of the modern-day activity known as chair yoga. It has been modified to cater to the requirements of older persons, who may have trouble doing conventional yoga postures due to physical restrictions or may not be able to perform as many poses as younger people.

In chair yoga, a chair is used as a prop to help support the body and guide the practitioner into the correct alignment of the postures. Because of this, a greater number of individuals, particularly those who have mobility impairments, arthritis, or balance problems, will be able to use it.

In healthcare settings such as rehabilitation and physical therapy, as well as in senior centers and assisted living facilities, chair yoga is a common form of exercise. It is also a common habit among senior citizens who want to enhance their general health and well-being while at the same time preserving their freedom.

Benefits of Chair Yoga for Older People

Chair yoga provides its participants with a broad variety of health advantages. The following are some of the most important advantages:

Increased Flexibility and Range of Motion: The majority of the postures in chair yoga concentrate on stretching the muscles and joints, which may assist enhance flexibility and range of motion. This may be particularly helpful for senior people, who may have lost some of their flexibility as a result of age or inactivity, and who may benefit the most from this.

Strengthening of the Muscles and Joints: Many of the Chair Yoga Poses Place an Emphasis on Strengthening the Muscles and Joints. This may assist in improving balance and stability, hence decreasing the likelihood of experiencing falls.

Increased Stability and Balancing: Many of the postures in chair yoga incorporate balance exercises, which may assist to increase both stability and balance. This is of utmost significance for senior citizens, who may be at a larger risk of falling, as compared to younger people.

Chair yoğa incorporates breathing exercises, which may assist to enhance both lung function and general respiratory health. These activities also contribute to improved breathing. This is especially crucial for older persons, who may have trouble breathing as a result of their age or other health concerns.

Chair yoga incorporates a number of different relaxation methods, such as deep breathing, meditation, and visualization, which all work together to reduce stress. These strategies may help to alleviate feelings of stress and anxiety, as well as enhance general health and well-being.

Increased Opportunities for Socialization Because chair yoga courses are often conducted in groups, they may provide seniors the chance to interact with new people and deepen their connections with those they already know. This may be particularly helpful for elderly people who may be living alone or who don't engage in as many social activities as younger people.

CHAPTER TWO

Getting Started

Safety Considerations

When it comes to starting any exercise program, it is important to consult with a healthcare provider to ensure that the practice is appropriate for you. This is especially important for older adults who may have underlying health conditions or physical limitations. Your healthcare provider can advise you on any modifications or precautions that may be necessary to ensure your safety while practicing Chair Yoga.

It is also important to be aware of any warning signs or symptoms that may indicate that you should stop practicing. These include pain, dizziness, shortness of breath, or feelings of lightheadedness. If you experience any of these symptoms, stop practicing immediately and consult with your healthcare provider.

Equipment Needed

Chair Yoga is a practice that requires minimal equipment. The only equipment needed is a chair and comfortable clothing that allows for easy movement. The chair should be stable and sturdy, and able to support your weight. Some poses may also require a towel or blanket for added support.

It is important to make sure that the chair you choose is the right size and height for you. The seat of the chair should be at hip height, and your feet should be able to touch the ground comfortably. If the chair is too high, you may find it difficult to maintain proper alignment in the poses. If the chair is too low, you may find it difficult to rise from the seated position.

Setting Up Your Space

When setting up your space for Chair Yoga, it is important to choose a quiet, comfortable space where you will be undisturbed. Make sure that the chair is stable and that there is enough room to move around. The space should be well-ventilated and have natural light, if possible.

It is also important to consider the temperature of the room. Yoga should be practiced in a room that is not too hot or too cold, as this can be distracting and uncomfortable. A room temperature of around 68-72 degrees Fahrenheit is ideal.

It's also important to have a clear and open mind when starting your practice. It is important to let go of any expectations or judgments and approach the practice with a sense of curiosity and openness. Remember that Chair Yoga is a process of self-discovery, and that progress may be slow. Be patient and kind to yourself, and celebrate small victories along the way.

In addition, setting up a regular practice schedule can help to establish a routine and make it easier to stick to your practice. Whether it's practicing every day or a few times a week, finding a time that works best for you and making it a regular part of your schedule can help to make it a sustainable practice.

To begin slowly: You should start with a few fundamental positions, and as you grow more familiar with the practice, you should progressively increase the number of poses as well as the complexity of the postures.

Always keep in mind to pay attention to your body and avoid going above your capabilities.

Generally, older individuals may enhance their flexibility, strength, balance, and overall well-being by engaging in Chair Yoga, which is a practice that is both mild and effective. It is a technique with minimal impact that is readily adaptable to fulfill the requirements of those who have physical limitations.

The practice of Chair Yoga incorporates many relaxation methods, which, when practiced regularly, have the potential to lower levels of stress and promote mental health. In addition to this, it offers the possibility of engaging in social activities and making connections with others in a group environment.

Finding community centers, senior centers, and fitness clubs offer courses in chair yoga. If you're interested in taking one, check out your local community center. You may also locate lessons on the internet, or you can buy DVDs to watch at home to help you practice.

We strongly suggest that you give Chair Yoga a go so that you may see its many advantages for yourself. It is essential that we keep our independence and the capacity to carry out the tasks of daily living as we become older.

Chair yoga has the potential to play a big part in assisting older persons in accomplishing this objective. The regular practice of Chair Yoga helps develop flexibility, strength, and balance, all of which are needed for carrying out day-to-day tasks such as walking, climbing stairs, and getting in and out of chairs.

Also, the regular use of relaxation methods, such as taking slow, deep breaths and meditating, may help to lessen feelings of tension and anxiety, which, in turn, can help one become better able to deal with the pressures and stresses of everyday life.

Chair yoga, when practiced on a consistent basis, may assist seniors in maintaining their independence, improving their general health and well-being, and leading lives that are richer and more satisfying.

CHAPTER THREE

Breathing Techniques for Chair Yoga

Breathing is an essential aspect of yoga practice, and it is even more important for older adults who may have respiratory issues. The practice of yoga breathing, also known as pranayama, can help seniors improve their lung capacity, reduce stress, and increase overall well-being. In this chapter, we will explore different types of breathing techniques that are suitable for chair yoga practice and their origins.

Diaphragmatic Breathing

Diaphragmatic breathing, also known as abdominal breathing, is a technique in which one focuses on expanding the diaphragm to draw air into the lungs.

This type of breathing is considered the most natural and efficient way of breathing as it engages the entire respiratory system, including the diaphragm, intercostal muscles, and abdominal muscles. The technique helps seniors increase their lung capacity and improve their overall breathing pattern.

Origination: Diaphragmatic breathing has been used in yoga and other forms of traditional medicine for thousands of years. The technique is believed to have originated in ancient India and was used as a tool for spiritual and physical well-being. In yoga, diaphragmatic breathing is considered one of the most basic and essential techniques for pranayama practice.

Ujjayi Breathing

Ujjayi breathing, also known as "victorious breath," is a technique in which one inhales and exhales through the nose while slightly constricting the back of the throat. The technique creates a soothing and calming sound, similar to the sound of ocean waves. Ujjayi breathing is believed to help seniors reduce stress, and anxiety, and improve their overall well-being.

Origination: Ujjayi breathing is an ancient technique that originated in India and is an integral part of the Hatha yoga practice. The technique is believed to have been passed down through generations of yogis and is considered one of the most basic pranayama techniques. The practice of ujjayi breathing is said to help regulate the mind and body, and it is considered to be a powerful tool for meditation and relaxation.

Nadi Shodhana Breathing

Nadi Shodhana breathing, also known as alternate nostril breathing, is a technique in which one alternately blocks and releases the flow of air through the nostrils. The technique is believed to balance the energy flow in the body and improve overall well-being. It is particularly helpful for seniors who may have respiratory issues or chronic stress.

Origination: Nadi Shodhana breathing is an ancient technique that originated in India and is an integral part of the Hatha yoga practice. The technique is believed to have been passed down through generations of yogis and is considered one of the most powerful pranayama techniques.

The practice of Nadi Shodhana breathing is said to balance the energy flow in the body, which can lead to improved physical and mental health.

These ancient techniques, which have been passed down through generations of yogis, are particularly beneficial for seniors as they can be easily practiced while seated in a chair. Incorporating these techniques into a regular chair yoga practice can bring about positive changes in the seniors' overall health and quality of life.

CHAPTER FOUR

Basic Chair Yoga Poses

It is crucial to have an understanding of the history of this one-of-a-kind kind of yoga before delving into the many positions that are a part of Chair Yoga.

Traditional yoga techniques have been reimagined in the form of chair yoga, which enables practitioners to carry out yoga postures either seated or standing with the use of a chair. This kind of yoga is very helpful for those who are healing from injuries or operations, as well as for elderly persons, people who have mobility or balance concerns, and anyone who is having trouble staying balanced.

The use of a chair as a prop not only makes it possible to do yoga postures in an atmosphere that is safe and stable, but it also makes it possible to provide extra support and aid to those who may need it.

The fundamental poses of Chair Yoga consist of a number of sitting and standing positions that aim to increase the practitioner's flexibility, balance, and a general sense of well-being. Because they may be adjusted to meet the unique requirements and capabilities of each person, these yoga positions are suitable for practitioners of varying degrees of physical fitness.

The sitting cat-cow posture, the seated downward-facing dog pose, the seated mountain pose, the seated forward bend, and the seated twist are all examples of frequent fundamental Chair Yoga poses. These positions are designed to improve total body alignment and balance while also extending and strengthening the hips, shoulders, and spine.

Once your physician has given you the green light to begin your practice, it is important to do so gradually. When you commit to practicing on a consistent basis, you will start to see good changes in both your body and your mind. Keep in mind that the process is just as essential as the final goal when it comes to chair yoga.

A. Seated Cat-Cow

The seated cat-cow pose is a simple yet effective pose that can be done in a chair to improve flexibility and mobility in the spine.

To begin, sit comfortably on the edge of the chair with your feet flat on the ground. Place your hands on your knees and take a deep breath in. As you exhale, round your spine forward, tucking your chin to your chest and bringing your shoulders forward. This is the cat position.

On the next inhale, arch your back and lift your head and shoulders. This is the cow position. Repeat this movement, alternating between cat and cow, for several deep breaths. This pose can help to stretch and strengthen the spine, as well as improve flexibility in the neck and shoulders.

Modification: If you have difficulty reaching your arms up toward the ceiling, you can keep your hands on your knees.

Variation: To add an extra challenge, try lifting your heels off the floor as you reach your arms up toward the ceiling.

B. Seated Downward Facing Dog

The seated downward-facing dog pose is a modified version of the traditional yoga pose and can be done in a chair to improve flexibility and strength in the upper body.

To begin, sit on the edge of the chair with your feet flat on the ground. Place your hands on the chair seat on either side of your hips and lift your hips up and back, bringing your body into an inverted 'V' shape.

Press your hands firmly into the chair seat and engage your core. Hold the pose for several deep breaths, then release. This pose can help to stretch and strengthen the shoulders, arms, and spine, as well as improve flexibility in the hips.

Modification: If you have difficulty reaching your heels down toward the floor, you can place a pillow or cushion under your heels for support.

Variation: To add an extra challenge, try lifting one leg off the floor and balancing on one leg.

C. Seated Mountain Pose

The seated mountain pose is a simple yet effective pose that can be done in a chair to improve posture and balance.

To begin, sit comfortably on the edge of the chair with your feet flat on the ground. Sit up tall and bring your shoulders back and down, engaging your core.

Lift your arms up overhead and interlace your fingers, pressing your palms together. Gaze forward and hold the pose for several deep breaths. This pose can help to improve posture, balance, and overall body alignment, as well as strengthen the core and upper body.

Modification: If you have difficulty sitting up tall, you can place a pillow or cushion behind your back for support.

Variation: To add an extra challenge, try lifting your arms toward the ceiling while maintaining your seated mountain pose.

D. Seated Forward Bend

The seated forward bend is a simple yet effective pose that can be done in a chair to improve flexibility in the hamstrings and lower back.

To begin, sit comfortably on the edge of the chair with your feet flat on the ground. Sit up tall and bring your shoulders back and down.

Reach forward, keeping your back straight and your head lifted, and place your hands on your feet or the ground in front of you. Hold the pose for several deep breaths, then release. This pose can help to stretch and release tension in the lower back and hamstrings, as well as improve overall flexibility.

Modification: If you have difficulty reaching your toes, you can place a pillow or cushion on your lap for support.

Variation: To add an extra challenge, try reaching your arms forward towards your toes without holding on to your knees.

E. Seated Twist

The seated twist is a simple yet effective pose that can be done in a chair to improve flexibility and mobility in the spine. To begin, sit comfortably on the edge of the chair with your feet flat on the ground. Sit up tall and bring your shoulders back and down.

Place your right hand on the back of the chair and your left hand on your right knee. Twist your torso to the right, keeping your shoulders back and down, and hold the pose for several deep breaths.

Release and repeat on the other side. This pose can help to stretch and release tension in the spine and improve mobility in the shoulders and hips.

Modification: If you have difficulty twisting your torso, you can place a pillow or cushion behind your back for support.

Variation: To add an extra challenge, try reaching your opposite arm behind you without holding on to the chair.

F. Seated Chair Pose

To begin, sit in a chair with your feet flat on the floor and your hands resting on your knees. Inhale and lift your arms up towards the ceiling, coming into a chair pose. Exhale and release. Repeat for 5-8 breaths.

Modification: If you have difficulty lifting your arms, you can place a pillow or cushion under your arms for support.

Variation: To add an extra challenge, try lifting one leg off the chair and balancing on one leg.

G. Seated Easy Pose

To begin, sit in a chair with your feet flat on the floor and your hands resting on your knees. Inhale and lift your arms up towards the ceiling, coming into an easy pose. Exhale and release. Repeat for 5-8 breaths.

Modification: If you have difficulty lifting your arms, you can place a pillow or cushion under your arms for support.

Variation: To add an extra challenge, try lifting one leg off the chair and balancing on one leg.

H. Seated Cobra Pose

To begin, sit in a chair with your feet flat on the floor and your hands resting on your knees. Inhale and lift your chest, coming into a cobra pose. Exhale and release. Repeat for 5-8 breaths.

Modification: If you have difficulty lifting your chest, you can place a pillow or cushion under your lower back for support.

Variation: To add an extra challenge, try lifting one leg off the chair and balancing on one leg.

I. Seated Eagle Pose

To begin, sit in a chair with your feet flat on the floor and your hands resting on your knees. Inhale and lift your arms up towards the ceiling, coming into an eagle pose. Exhale and release. Repeat for 5-8 breaths.

Modification: If you have difficulty lifting your arms, you can place a pillow or cushion under your arms for support.

Variation: To add an extra challenge, try lifting one leg off the chair and balancing on one leg.

J. Seated Half Moon Pose

To begin, sit in a chair with your feet flat on the floor and your hands resting on your knees. Slowly twist your torso to the right, placing your left hand on the back of the chair and extending your right arm towards the ceiling. Hold for 5-8 breaths before switching sides.

Modification: If you have difficulty twisting your torso, you can place a pillow or cushion behind your lower back for support.

Variation: To add an extra challenge, try lifting one leg off the chair and balancing on one leg while in the half-moon pose.

L. Seated Half Lord of the Fishes Pose

To begin, sit in a chair with your feet flat on the floor and your hands resting on your knees. Slowly twist your torso to the right and bring your left elbow to the outside of your right knee while your right hand extends toward the ceiling. Hold for 5-8 breaths before switching sides.

Modification: If you have difficulty twisting your torso, you can place a pillow or cushion behind your lower back for support.

Variation: To add an extra challenge, try lifting one leg off the chair and balancing on one leg while in the half lord of the fishes pose.

M. Seated Head-to-Knee Pose

To begin, sit in a chair with your feet flat on the floor and your hands resting on your knees. Slowly bend one leg and bring the heel towards your inner thigh, extending the other leg straight out in front of you. Bring your head towards your bent knee and hold for 5-8 breaths before switching sides.

Modification: If you have difficulty reaching your head towards your knee, you can place a pillow or cushion under your bent knee for support.

Variation: To add an extra challenge, try lifting one arm toward the ceiling while in the head-to-knee pose.

N. Seated Wheel Pose

To begin, sit in a chair with your feet flat on the floor and your hands resting on your knees. Slowly lift your body off the chair by placing your hands behind your head and extending your legs straight out in front of you. Hold for 5-8 breaths.

Modification: If you have difficulty lifting your body off the chair, you can place a pillow or cushion under your head for support.

Variation: To add an extra challenge, try lifting both legs off the chair while in the wheel pose.

O. Seated Hand-to-Big-Toe Pose

To begin, sit in a chair with your feet flat on the floor and your hands resting on your knees. Slowly extend one leg straight out in front of you and bring your hand towards the big toe of that leg. Hold for 5-8 breaths before switching sides.

Modification: If you have difficulty reaching your hand to your big toe, you can place a pillow or cushion under your extended leg for support.

Variation: To add an extra challenge, try lifting the other arm towards the ceiling while in the hand-to-big-toe pose.

P. Seated Sun Salutation

To begin, sit in a chair with your feet flat on the floor and your hands resting on your knees. Take a deep breath in and raise your arms above your head, reaching towards the sky. As you exhale, lower your arms back down to your sides. Repeat this sequence for 5-8 rounds.

Modification: If you have difficulty raising your arms above your head, you can keep your hands resting on your knees or bring them to your chest.

Variation: To add an extra challenge, try adding a twist to each round of the sun salutation by bringing one hand to the opposite knee as you exhale.

Note: It's important to remember that modifications and variations are offered to cater to individual abilities and should be used as necessary. Yoga practice should be comfortable and enjoyable, listen to your body and never push beyond your limits.

You may enhance your flexibility, balance, and general quality of life by including these fundamental postures in your daily practice. Keep in mind that the goal is not the point of this adventure.

Take everything slowly, pay attention to what your body is telling you, and be patient with yourself. It is not about reaching perfection; rather, the focus should be on making progress. You will be able to carry out your day-to-day tasks with more ease and freedom after you develop consistent practice.

You will also begin to notice good changes in both your body and your mind as a result of these changes. Always keep in mind that the journey is the goal while practicing Chair Yoga.

CHAPTER FIVE

Intermediate Chair Yoga Poses

This chapter will take us further into the practice of chair yoga by introducing us to several positions that are considered to be intermediate.

Your balance, flexibility, and strength will all be tested in unique ways as you go through these yoga positions, which will also assist you to go deeper into your practice. The sat warrior posture, the seated triangle pose, the seated half lotus stance, the seated chair balancing pose and the seated camel pose are going to be our primary focuses.

Each posture will be broken down into its component movements in a step-by-step manner, and adaptations and variants will be provided for individuals who may have difficulties doing specific motions. Always be sure to pay attention to what your body is telling you and resist the urge to test your boundaries.

A. Seated Warrior Pose

The seated warrior pose is a great way to strengthen the legs, arms, and core, while also stretching the hips and shoulders.

To begin, sit in a chair with your feet flat on the floor, hip-distance apart. Place your hands on the arms of the chair, and lift up out of your seat, engaging your core. Bring your left leg to the front of the chair, with your knee bent at a 90-degree angle.

Keep your right leg behind you, with your heel on the floor. Reach your arms up towards the ceiling, and look up towards your hands. Hold for 5-8 breaths, then release and repeat on the other side.

Modification: If you have difficulty lifting out of your seat, you can place a pillow or cushion behind your back to prop yourself up.

Variation: To add an extra challenge, try lifting the back leg off the floor and balancing on one leg.

B. Seated Triangle Pose

The seated triangle pose is a great way to stretch the sides of the body and improve balance.

To begin, sit in a chair with your feet flat on the floor, hip-distance apart. Place your left hand on the left arm of the chair, and reach your right arm up towards the ceiling.

Slowly twist your torso to the right, reaching your right arm towards the back of the chair. Keep your left hand on the chair for support, and hold for 5-8 breaths. Release and repeat on the other side.

Modification: If you have difficulty twisting your torso, you can keep your right hand on your right knee, and reach your left hand towards the back of the chair.

Variation: To add an extra challenge, try reaching your right arm towards the back of the chair without holding on to the chair.

C. Seated Half Lotus

The seated half lotus pose is a great way to stretch the hips and improve flexibility.

To begin, sit in a chair with your feet flat on the floor, hip-distance apart. Bring your left foot up to rest on top of your right thigh, with your heel as close to your hip as possible. Hold on to the chair for support, and hold for 5-8 breaths. Release and repeat on the other side.

Modification: If you have difficulty lifting your foot up to your thigh, you can place a strap or belt around your foot, and use it to pull your foot up towards your thigh.

Variation: To add an extra challenge, try lifting your right arm up towards the ceiling, and reaching it over your head.

D. Seated Chair Balance

The seated chair balance is a great way to improve balance and focus.

To begin, sit in a chair with your feet flat on the floor, hip-distance apart. Place your hands on the arms of the chair, and lift up out of your seat, engaging your core.

Slowly lift your right foot off the floor, and bring it to rest on top of your left thigh. Hold for 5-8 breaths, then release and repeat on the other side.

Modification: If you have difficulty lifting your foot off the floor, you can place a pillow or cushion under your foot for support.

Variation: To add an extra challenge, try lifting your arms up towards the ceiling while maintaining your balance on one foot.

E. Seated Camel Pose

The seated camel pose is a great way to stretch the spine and open the chest.

To begin, sit in a chair with your feet flat on the floor, hip-distance apart. Place your hands on the back of the chair, and lift up out of your seat, engaging your core.

Slowly lean back, reaching your hands towards your heels. Keep your head and neck in a neutral position, and hold for 5-8 breaths. Release and repeat as desired.

Modification: If you have difficulty leaning back, you can place a pillow or cushion behind your back for support.

Variation: To add an extra challenge, try reaching your hands behind your heels without holding on to the chair.

F. Seated Crescent Pose

To begin, sit in a chair with your feet flat on the floor and your hands resting on your knees. Slowly lift one leg

off the chair and extend it straight behind you while keeping your torso facing forward and your arms extended in front of you. Slowly lift your arms up towards the ceiling and lean your torso forward. Hold for 5-8 breaths before switching sides.

Modification: If you have difficulty lifting your leg, you can place a pillow or cushion under your lifted leg for support.

Variation: To add an extra challenge, try lifting both legs off the chair while in the crescent pose.

G. Seated Side Angle Pose

To begin, sit in a chair with your feet flat on the floor and your hands resting on your knees. Slowly twist your torso to the right and extend your left arm towards the back of the chair while your right arm extends towards the ceiling.

Slowly lift your left leg off the chair and place your foot on the chair beside your right thigh. Hold for 5-8 breaths before switching sides.

Modification: If you have difficulty lifting your leg, you can place a pillow or cushion under your lifted leg for support.

Variation: To add an extra challenge, try lifting both arms up towards the ceiling while in the side-angle pose.

H. Seated Chair Bow Pose

To begin, sit in a chair with your feet flat on the floor and your hands resting on your knees. Slowly bring your left ankle to your right knee and extend your left arm towards the back of the chair while your right arm extends towards the ceiling. Slowly lean your torso forward and hold for 5-8 breaths before switching sides.

Modification: If you have difficulty leaning forward, you can keep your spine straight and bring your hands to your ankle instead of reaching them towards the back of the chair.

Variation: To add an extra challenge, try lifting both arms up towards the ceiling while in the chair bow pose.

I. Seated Chair Pigeon Pose

To begin, sit in a chair with your feet flat on the floor and your hands resting on your knees. Slowly bring your left ankle to your right knee and extend your left arm towards the back of the chair while your right arm extends towards the ceiling.

Slowly lean your torso forward and extend your left leg straight out behind you. Hold for 5-8 breaths before switching sides.

Modification: If you have difficulty sitting in the full king pigeon pose, you can place a pillow or cushion under your lifted hip for support and keep your extended leg bent.

Variation: To add an extra challenge, try lifting both arms up towards the ceiling while in the chair king pigeon pose.

Note: It is important to remember to breathe deeply and focus on your breath throughout each pose. This will help to calm your mind and increase the effectiveness of the poses.

In addition, it's important to always use a sturdy chair that can support your weight and is comfortable to sit on. Avoid using a chair with wheels or one that is too soft or too hard.

You may take your practice to the next level by using these chair yoga positions that are considered to be intermediate.

They will provide you with fresh challenges in terms of your balance, flexibility, and strength, and they will assist you in going deeper into your yoga practice. You will eventually be able to do these postures with ease if you start gently, implement changes as necessary, and have time and patience on your side.

Lastly, it's important to be patient with yourself and not push yourself too hard. Yoga is a practice that takes time and dedication to master. As you progress, you will be

able to hold poses for longer periods of time and even attempt more advanced poses.

CHAPTER SIX

Advanced Chair Yoga Poses

As we progress through our yoga practice, we may find ourselves ready to take on more challenging poses. The advanced chair yoga poses in this chapter are designed to challenge your balance, flexibility, and strength in new ways.

However, it's important to remember that these poses are considered advanced for a reason, and they should only be attempted by those who have a solid foundation in basic and intermediate chair yoga poses. It is also crucial to listen to your body and never push beyond your limits.

A. Seated Tree Pose

The seated tree pose is a great way to challenge your balance and stability.

To begin, sit in a chair with your feet flat on the floor, hip-distance apart. Bring your right foot up and place it on the left thigh, pressing the sole of the foot into the thigh.

Bring your hands together in a prayer position and bring them to your chest. Hold for 5-8 breaths, then release and repeat on the other side.

Modification: If you have difficulty balancing on one foot, you can place a pillow or cushion under your foot for support.

Variation: To add an extra challenge, try lifting your arms up towards the ceiling while maintaining your balance on one foot.

B. Seated Warrior II

The seated warrior II is a great way to challenge your strength and stability.

To begin, sit in a chair with your feet flat on the floor, hip-distance apart. Bring your right foot up and place it on the floor next to your left knee.

Bring your hands up to shoulder height and look over your right hand. Hold for 5-8 breaths, then release and repeat on the other side.

Modification: If you have difficulty lifting your foot off the floor, you can place a pillow or cushion under your foot for support.

Variation: To add an extra challenge, try lifting your arms up towards the ceiling while maintaining your balance on one foot.

C. Seated Half Lord of the Fishes

The seated half lord of the fishes is a great way to challenge your flexibility and stability.

To begin, sit in a chair with your feet flat on the floor, hip-distance apart. Bring your right foot up and place it on the left thigh, pressing the sole of the foot into the thigh.

Bring your left elbow to the outside of your right knee and twist your torso towards the right. Hold for 5-8 breaths, then release and repeat on the other side.

Modification: If you have difficulty twisting your torso, you can place a pillow or cushion behind your back for support.

Variation: To add an extra challenge, try reaching your opposite arm behind you without holding on to the chair.

D. Seated Head-to-Knee Pose

The seated head-to-knee pose is a great way to challenge your flexibility and stability.

To begin, sit in a chair with your feet flat on the floor, hip-distance apart. Bring your right foot up and place it on the left thigh, pressing the sole of the foot into the thigh.

Bring your left elbow to the outside of your right knee and twist your torso towards the right. Hold for 5-8 breaths, then release and repeat on the other side.

Modification: If you have difficulty touching your toes, you can place a pillow or cushion on your lap for support.

Variation: To add an extra challenge, try reaching your arms forward towards your toes without holding on to your knees.

E. Seated Eagle Pose

The seated eagle pose is a great way to challenge your flexibility and stability.

To begin, sit in a chair with your feet flat on the floor, hip-distance apart. Bring your right foot up and place it on top of the left thigh. Bring your left arm under your right arm and twist your hands together. Hold for 5-8 breaths, then release and repeat on the other side.

Modification: If you have difficulty crossing your legs or twisting your arms, you can place a pillow or cushion under your legs for support.

Variation: To add an extra challenge, try lifting your arms up toward the ceiling while maintaining your eagle pose.

F. Seated Half Handstand

To begin, sit in a chair and place your hands on the seat beside you, fingers pointing towards the back of the chair. Press into your hands and lift your hips off the chair, coming into a half-handstand position. Hold for 5-8 breaths.

Modification: If you have difficulty lifting your hips off the chair, you can place a pillow or cushion under your hips for support.

Variation: To add an extra challenge, try lifting one leg off the chair and balancing on one leg.

G. Seated Crow Pose

To begin, sit in a chair and place your hands on the seat beside you, fingers pointing towards the back of the chair. Bend your knees and bring your shins parallel to the floor. Shift your weight forward, lift your hips off the chair, and bring your knees to rest on the back of your upper arms. Hold for 5-8 breaths.

Modification: If you have difficulty lifting your hips off the chair, you can place a pillow or cushion under your hips for support.

Variation: To add an extra challenge, try lifting one leg off the chair and balancing on one leg.

H. Seated Wheel Pose

To begin, sit in a chair and place your hands on the seat beside you, fingers pointing towards the back of the chair. Bring your feet to rest on top of the chair seat, and press into your hands and feet, lifting your hips off the chair and coming into a wheel pose. Hold for 5-8 breaths

Modification: If you have difficulty lifting your hips off the chair, you can place a pillow or cushion under your hips for support.

Variation: To add an extra challenge, try lifting one leg off the chair and balancing on one leg.

I. Seated Headstand

To begin, sit in a chair and place your hands on the seat beside you, fingers pointing towards the back of the chair. Place the top of your head on the seat of the chair and walk your feet towards your head. Press into your hands and lift your hips off the chair, coming into a headstand position. Hold for 5-8 breaths.

Modification: If you have difficulty lifting your hips off the chair, you can place a pillow or cushion under your hips for support.

Variation: To add an extra challenge, try lifting one leg off the chair and balancing on one leg.

J. Seated Lotus Pose

To begin, sit in a chair and bring your right foot up to rest on your left thigh. Bring your left foot up and place it on top of your right thigh. Bring your hands to your heart in a prayer position and hold for 5-8 breaths. Repeat on the other side.

Modification: If you have difficulty crossing your legs, you can place a pillow or cushion under your legs for support.

Variation: To add an extra challenge, try lifting your arms up toward the ceiling while maintaining your lotus pose.

CHAPTER SEVEN

Chair Yoga Sequences

In the next section, we will investigate chair yoga sequences that have been particularly constructed for the morning, afternoon, and evening.

The body has certain requirements at various times of the day, and these sequences are designed to meet those requirements. The morning sequence is intended to rouse the body, establish a constructive mood for the day, and relieve stress that may have built up during the previous night's sleep.

The purpose of the afternoon sequence is to relieve the stress that might build up in the body as a result of prolonged periods of sitting, as well as to stretch and strengthen the body.

The goal of the evening sequence is to relax the mind and body in preparation for a pleasant night's sleep and to let go of any tension or stress that has built up during the day.

You may enhance both your physical and emotional well-being by making chair yoga a regular part of your practice and reaping the benefits of doing so.

A. *Morning Sequence*

Sitting Tall: Start the day by sitting up straight in your chair with both feet flat on the floor. Take a deep breath in and lift your arms above your head, stretching as high as you can.

Exhale and release your arms back down to your sides. Repeat this movement for several breaths. This simple exercise can help wake up your body and set a positive tone for the day ahead.

Shoulder Rolls: Sitting up straight, inhale and lift your shoulders towards your ears. Exhale and roll your shoulders back and down.

Repeat this movement for several breaths. This exercise can help release tension in the shoulders, which can often accumulate overnight.

Neck Stretch: Sitting up straight, inhale, and bring your right ear towards your right shoulder. Exhale and release.

Inhale and bring your left ear towards your left shoulder. Exhale and release. Repeat this movement for several breaths, being sure to keep your shoulders relaxed.

This exercise can help release tension in the neck, which is common after a night's sleep.

Spinal Twist: Sitting up straight, inhale and twist your torso to the right. Place your left hand on the back of the chair and your right hand on your right knee.

Exhale and release. Inhale and twist your torso to the left. Place your right hand on the back of the chair and your left hand on your left knee. Exhale and release. Repeat this movement for several breaths. This exercise can help release tension in the spine, which can also accumulate overnight.

Seated Sun Salutation: Sitting up straight, inhale, and lift your arms above your head. Exhale and bend forward, reaching for your toes. Inhale and sit up straight.

Exhale and twist your torso to the right. Inhale and release. Exhale and twist your torso to the left. Inhale and release.

Repeat this movement for several breaths. This exercise can help wake up your body, stretch your muscles, and get your blood flowing.

B. Afternoon Sequence

Seated Cat-Cow: Sit up straight in your chair, with your feet flat on the floor. Inhale and arch your back, lifting your chin and tailbone towards the ceiling.

Exhale and round your back, tucking your chin towards your chest. Repeat this movement for several breaths. This exercise can help release tension in the back, which can accumulate from sitting for long periods of time.

Seated Forward Bend: Sit up straight in your chair, with your feet flat on the floor. Inhale and lift your arms up above your head. Exhale and bend forward, reaching for your toes. Inhale and release. Repeat this movement for several breaths. This exercise can help release tension in the back and stretch the hamstrings.

Seated Warrior: Sit up straight in your chair, with your feet flat on the floor. Inhale and lift your arms up above your head. Exhale and twist your torso to the right, placing your left hand on the back of the chair and your right hand on your right knee. Inhale and release.

Exhale and twist your torso to the left, placing your right hand on the back of the chair and your left hand on your left knee. Inhale and release. Repeat this movement for several breaths. This exercise can help release tension in the back and stretch the hips.

Seated Eagle: Sit up straight in your chair, with your feet flat on the floor. Cross your right thigh over your left thigh, and cross your right arm over your left arm. Inhale and lift your arms up above your head.

Exhale and release. Repeat this movement for several breaths. This exercise can help release tension in the shoulders and stretch the hips.

Seated Meditation: Sit up straight in your chair, with your feet flat on the floor. Close your eyes and focus on your breath. Allow your mind to clear and release any tension or stress.

Sit in this position for as long as you feel comfortable, and then slowly open your eyes when you are ready to return to your day.

C. Evening Sequence

Seated Relaxation: Sit up straight in your chair, with your feet flat on the floor. Close your eyes and focus on your breath. Allow your body to relax and release any tension or stress. Sit in this position for as long as you feel comfortable, and then slowly open your eyes when you are ready to end your practice.

Seated Mindfulness: Sit up straight in your chair, with your feet flat on the floor. Close your eyes and focus on your breath. Allow your mind to clear and release any thoughts or worries. Sit in this position for as long as you feel comfortable, and then slowly open your eyes when you are ready to end your practice.

Seated Yoga Nidra: Sit up straight in your chair, with your feet flat on the floor. Close your eyes and focus on your breath.

Allow your mind and body to relax, sinking deeper and deeper into a state of complete relaxation.

During this practice, you can guide yourself through a body scan, focusing on each part of your body and releasing any tension or stress. This practice can help prepare your mind and body for a restful night's sleep.

Seated Savasana: Sit up straight in your chair, with your feet flat on the floor. Close your eyes and focus on your breath. Allow your body to relax completely, letting go of any tension or stress. Sit in this position for several minutes, and then slowly open your eyes when you are ready to end your practice.

The sequences provided in this chapter can help improve flexibility, balance, and overall well-being. Whether you're a beginner or an advanced practitioner, these sequences can be adapted to suit your needs and help you maintain a consistent yoga practice.

Remember, consistency is key, and try to practice regularly, whether it's in the morning, afternoon, or evening, you will see the benefits of chair yoga in no time.

CHAPTER EIGHT

Special Considerations

As we age, our bodies may experience changes in mobility and flexibility. It's important to remember that yoga is not a one-size-fits-all practice and should be adapted to suit the individual's needs.

In this chapter, we will explore special considerations for chair yoga in depth, including modifying poses for limited mobility, adapting poses for specific conditions, and incorporating props. By understanding and implementing these modifications, older adults can continue to practice yoga safely and comfortably.

A. Modifying Poses for Limited Mobility

It's important to remember that not all poses can be done by everyone. As we age, our bodies may experience changes in mobility and flexibility, and it's important to be mindful of these changes and make modifications as needed.

For example, if you have difficulty reaching your toes, you can modify the seated forward bend by placing a yoga block under your hands. This will allow you to still maintain the stretch in the hamstrings and lower back without overstretching or straining the back.

Another modification for seated forward bend could be to bend the knees and hold the feet or ankle instead of the toes. This will allow for a safe and comfortable stretch.

If you have difficulty lifting your arms above your head, you can modify the seated sun salutation by keeping your arms at your sides. This modification allows you to still engage the upper body and shoulders while avoiding any discomfort or strain in the shoulders.

It's also important to pay attention to the alignment of the spine while practicing seated poses, especially if you have limited mobility in the spine. Keeping the spine straight and aligned while practicing seated poses can help prevent strain and discomfort.

Remember, always listen to your body, and don't push yourself beyond your limits. It's important to move slowly and be mindful of your breath.

B. Adapting Poses for Specific Conditions

Certain conditions, such as arthritis or osteoporosis, may require additional modifications to poses. For example, if you have arthritis, it's important to avoid poses that put pressure on the joints.

Poses such as seated forward bend and seated twist should be modified to prevent any discomfort or pain in the joints.

If you have osteoporosis, it's important to avoid poses that involve twisting or bending forward, as these poses can put pressure on the spine and increase the risk of fractures. Poses such as seated forward bend and seated twist should be modified by keeping the spine straight and aligned, and avoiding any twisting or bending forward.

It's important to consult with your doctor or a qualified yoga instructor to determine which poses are appropriate for you and what modifications should be made. They can help you create a practice that is safe and effective for your specific condition.

C. Incorporating Props

Props can be used to make poses more accessible and comfortable. For example, a yoga block can be used to rest your hands during a seated forward bend, or a blanket can be used to cushion your knees during a seated twist. These props can help to reduce the risk of injury and make poses more accessible.

A chair itself can also be used as a prop, for example using it for balance during standing poses. Holding onto the back of the chair for balance during standing poses such as warrior 2 can help to increase stability and reduce the risk of falling.

It's also important to incorporate props such as straps or scarves to help reach and hold onto during seated forward bends and other seated poses to help maintain proper alignment and avoid overstretching.

Always keep in mind the importance of having patience with yourself and not pushing yourself beyond your capabilities. You will start to feel the advantages of chair yoga almost immediately if you practice it regularly and have patience.

If you are interested in increasing your flexibility, balance, or general well-being, chair yoga may be able to assist you in accomplishing your objectives in a method that is both safe and pleasant.

It is essential to keep in mind that yoga is not a practice that can be applied universally and that it must be modified to meet the requirements of the practitioner.

You may continue to practice yoga in a safe and comfortable manner as long as you pay attention to your body, pay attention to the restrictions it presents, and make adaptations as necessary.

CHAPTER NINE

Conclusion

This is the last chapter, and in it, we will go further into the numerous advantages of chair yoga for older people, promote the continuous practice, and present extra resources for those who are wishing to expand their current yoga practice.

In addition to this, we will talk about the significance of maintaining a healthy lifestyle as we get older and the positive effects that regular chair yoga practice can have on one's general health and well-being.

By the time you reach the conclusion of this chapter, you will have a deeper comprehension of the plethora of advantages that chair yoga provides, as well as the constructive influence that it may have on your life.

A. Summary of Benefits

There are a lot of different and far-reaching advantages that older folks may get from doing chair yoga. Chair yoga, when practiced on a regular basis, may lead to improvements in a person's flexibility, balance, and strength.

Regularly engaging in yoga practice may assist people of a certain age to improve their posture and alignment, both of which are important factors in lowering the probability of experiencing injuries and falling down.

Enhancing one's flexibility and balance may also contribute to an increase in one's mobility and level of independence, which in turn enables older persons to continue to participate in their everyday activities without much difficulty.

Chair yoga, in addition to its numerous positive effects on the body, it has a significant positive impact on the mind and the emotions.

Yoga's emphasis on contemplative practices and mindfulness may make it an effective tool for relieving stress and anxiety while also fostering feelings of serenity and general well-being. In addition to these benefits, yoga has been shown to help enhance the quality of sleep, raise mood, and even reduce blood pressure.

Because it is a low-impact kind of exercise, chair yoga is a sort of physical activity that may be done by older persons who have mobility issues or other types of physical restrictions.

It is a kind of exercise that is risk-free and easy on the joints, and it can be adjusted to meet the requirements of the person doing it, even if they have a chronic illness such as osteoporosis or arthritis, or if they have restricted mobility.

B. Encouragement to Continue Practicing

As we've seen, older folks may benefit from and easily participate in chair yoga, which is an accessible type of exercise.

The accumulation of positive effects on one's body, mind, and emotions may be the result of consistent practice.

We strongly recommend that you make chair yoga a regular part of your daily routine and that you perform the practice with patience and consistency.

Keep in mind that maintaining a consistent routine is essential for achieving success with any fitness regimen. It is essential to devote some portion of each day to deliberate practice, even if that time commitment is just brief in duration. You won't have to wait long until you feel the positive effects of chair yoga if you practice it regularly.

C. The Importance of Making Health a Priority

As we become older, it is imperative that we make maintaining our health and well-being a top concern.

Exercise on a regular basis, such as chair yoga, may assist to enhance the overall quality of life, as well as one's physical and mental health, as well as minimize the chance of developing chronic illnesses.

It is essential to keep in mind that the goal of maintaining a healthy lifestyle is not just to avoid becoming sick but also to improve one's quality of life and have fun.

A consistent practice of chair yoga may assist to enhance mood, raise energy levels, and create a feeling of well-being in addition to other potential benefits. We may continue to have an active and satisfying life as we become older if we make taking care of our health a top priority.

D. Additional Sources of Information

There is a large variety of materials accessible to assist you in developing your practice further if you so want. Chair yoga programs are often available in community centers and yoga studios, and many classes cater exclusively to senior citizens.

You can also find numerous videos and lessons online that are particularly dedicated to older persons and can walk you through different chair yoga sequences to help guide you through the practice.

E. The Final Thoughts

In conclusion, older folks may benefit from chair yoga since it is a kind of exercise that is not only approachable but also beneficial. It is possible, with consistent practice, to see improvements in flexibility, balance, and general well-being.

I have faith in you and your capacity to incorporate chair yoga into your daily routine, and I am certain that if you are patient and persistent, you will begin to experience the advantages of chair yoga in a very short amount of time.

Always keep in mind the importance of making your own health and well-being a top priority, and don't forget to look into other resources to expand your knowledge about chair yoga and the advantages it offers. It is important to remember to practice chair yoga on a daily basis in order to reap the advantages it has on your physical, mental, and emotional well-being.